MIGRAINE

Reset Your Brain

By

JASSICA ROW

Table of Contents

Chapter 1 5

What is migraine? 5

Chapter 2 8

Different types of migraines 8

Chapter 3 52

Four phases of an intermittent migraine.....52

Prodromal period....................................52

Aura phase 53

Headache period.....................................54

Postdrome phase 55

Chapter 4 56

SEX,GENDER AND MIGRAINE 56

Chapter 5 105

Theories concerning migraine pain............105

Chapter 6 109

Migraines diagnosis 109

Chapter 7 112

Acute Migraine...112

Chapter 8 116

Migraine in children 116

Chapter 9 135

MIGRAINE AND STRESS.............................135

Non-pharmacological approaches to the treatment of headaches in children and adolescents 156

Relaxation techniques............................158

Exercise 160

Acupuncture...160

Sleep..161

Chapter 11 164

Monitor Migraine...164

Chapter 1

What is migraine?

A migraine is more than just a bad headache. Compared to other headache syndromes, it is a crippling neurological illness with distinctive symptoms and therapeutic approaches. According to the American Migraine Foundation, at least 39 million Americans experience migraines; however, the actual number is likely higher because many sufferers do not obtain a proper diagnosis or treatment. The sixth most common disease in the world and a major contributor to disability, migraine causes severe personal and societal distress.

Migraine is a severe and chronically painful illness. Migraine sufferers will experience migraine attacks, which can involve the entire body.

- Headache,
- Vision difficulties, such as seeing flashing lights,
- Sensitivity to light, sounds, and odors,
- Fatigue,
- feeling unwell,

Different folks receive different symptoms. During a migraine attack, it may be impossible to function regularly.

Attacks of migraine typically last between four hours and three days. Some symptoms may begin approximately 24 hours before to the onset of head pain and last approximately 24 hours after the headache subsides. Most individuals experience no symptoms between migraine bouts.

Migraines are a type of recurrent headache. They induce moderate to severe throbbing or pulsating discomfort.

Typically, the pain is on one side of the head. Migraine is frequently characterized by throbbing pain in one area of the head for four to seventy-two hours. Some people experience as zigzag lines or flashing lights prior to or during a migraine.

Migraine is believed to impact more than 10% of the world's population, is most prevalent between the ages of 20 and 50. In a comprehensive survey conducted in the United States, 17.1% of women and 5.6% of males suffered migraine symptoms.

Chapter 2

Different types of migraines

With or without aura?

Migraine with aura, formerly known as "classical migraines," and migraine without aura are the two most common forms (previously known as "common migraines").

One type of migraine is a migraine aura without a headache. You can see dots, wavy lines, or flashing lights when you have an aura. Your face, arms, or hands could feel tingly or numb. But in contrast to other headaches, the aura doesn't come first.

Some people experience migraines of both types. They sometimes have an aura without a headache, but they might also have an aura followed by a headache.

Migraines can persist anywhere from four hours to a few days if untreated. Medication can either halt or prevent migraines. On this, your doctor can provide you advice.

You must receive follow-up care if you want to be healthy and happy. Remind yourself to keep all appointments, and call your doctor if something seems off. Along with keeping track of the prescriptions you are taking, you should be informed of the results of your tests.

What self-care techniques can you use at home?

> - If you've taken a prescription painkiller, don't go behind the wheel.
> - Remain in a quiet, dark room until your headache or aura goes away. Be sure to close your eyes. Try to relax or sleep. Avoid reading and watching television.
> - Apply a cool, wet cloth or a cold pack to the affected area for 10 to

20 minutes if you have a headache. Place a little piece of cloth between the skin and the cold pack.

➢ Apply a low-temperature heating pad or a warm, damp cloth to the affected area. This may aid in easing neck and shoulder stiffness.

➢ Have your neck and shoulders softly massaged.

➢ When utilizing medications, use caution. Take your medications as directed. If you think there could be a problem with your medication, call your doctor or the nurse call line. More details regarding the precise meds that your doctor has advised will be delivered to you.

➢ Avoid using painkillers too regularly. If you take headache medicine more than twice a week, speak with your doctor. Overdosing on painkillers might make headaches worse. These are referred to as headaches from drug misuse.

To avoid getting migraines

- ✓ Maintain a journal to track the origin of your headaches or auras. By preventing the triggers of migraines, they can be prevented. Each headache or aura should be noted along with its onset, duration, and accompanying symptoms.
- ✓ Note any additional symptoms that may have appeared along with the aura. Examples of these symptoms include nausea and sensitivity to loud noises or bright light, respectively. Note whether the headache or aura happened throughout your period. Make a list of all the aura's potential causes. Some foods (such as chocolate, cheese, and wine), odors, smoke, bright lights, stress, and sleep deprivation are triggers.
- ✓ Be sure to follow the directions on any medicine your doctor has recommended for your migraines. Only when you are experiencing a

migraine may you take a migraine medicine, and you should take a migraine medication every day to avoid migraines.

✓ Unless your doctor has told you otherwise, take any prescription migraine medicine at the first indication of an aura.

✓ Follow the directions on any migraine medicine that your doctor has recommended. If you think you might have a medication issue, go to your doctor.

✓ Create efficient coping strategies for stress. Most people have migraines during or right after stressful situations. Take into account methods for reducing stress including mindfulness and deep breathing.

✓ Get enough sleep and engage in regular exercise. But when exercising, don't expend too much effort. It might give you a headache.

- ✓ Consume regular meals and stay away from substances that frequently cause migraines. Among them are alcohol, particularly red wine and port, and chocolate. Migraines may be brought on by food additives like aspartame and monosodium glutamate (msg). Some food additives, including those in cold cuts, hot dogs, and bacon, pickled foods, and aged cheeses, can also cause cancer.
- ✓ Limit your intake of caffeine by avoiding soda, tea, and coffee. However, quitting coffee suddenly can result in headaches.
- ✓ Don't smoke, and don't let anyone else smoke around you. Consult your doctor about stop-smoking programmes and drugs if you need assistance quitting. These may improve your chances of successfully quitting.
- ✓ If you take birth control pills or hormone therapy, discuss it with

your doctor to determine whether they may be contributing to your migraines.

When should you get assistance?

You exhibit signs of a stroke. Here are a few instances:

- o An unexpected loss of sensation, tingling, strength, or range of motion in the face, arm, or leg, often on one side.
- o Sudden adjustments to vision.
- o Suddenly having trouble speaking.

People with both types of migraine are frequently permitted to take part in the same research trials, although migraine with aura has not been examined as thoroughly as migraine without aura.

The lower prevalence of migraines with aura and the challenges in studying the aura episode itself may both play a significant role in this.

Aura is rarely seen on computed tomography scans, despite the fact that patients with aura are more likely to be referred for the procedure because there is currently no viable way to predict or create the phenomenon.

Additionally, getting a scan during an aura is impossible due to its short lifespan (approximately 60 minutes).

White matter abnormalities were seen in patients with migraine four times more frequently than in the general population during imaging studies, however migraine with aura and migraine without aura showed similar structural changes to the brain.

Previous studies showed show differences in the blood flow dynamics between the two types of migraines.

However, studies have recently started to differentiate between migraines with and without aura, showing a number of other important findings:

• Compared to migraine without aura, which is more common, migraine with aura frequently has a more striking array of clinical indications.

• Compared to migraine without aura, migraine with aura is associated with a twofold increased risk of stroke.

• Imaging studies show that structural brain function impairments are more apparent in aura-associated headaches.

• The cerebral blood flow patterns of migraines with and without aura could differ.

• Acute and preventive therapies have quite different therapeutic outcomes.

Auras that accompany migraines may not be a singular entity, according to studies, but rather a diverse range of pathophysiological symptoms.

Protracted auras, manifestations with somatosensory, dysphasic, or motor characteristics, and those with a predominance of visual components are some examples of different manifestations.

The timing of the aura varies as well. The majority start before the pain of a migraine headache, but different types of migraines can also start at the same time or without a headache. While aura is present, attack triggers are less likely to be reported. These temporal discrepancies suggest that cortical spreading depression may contribute to aura, though not necessarily all migraines.

People who experience migraine and a cryptogenic stroke simultaneously are more likely (79%) to have patent foramen ovale, a congenital heart defect.

This gets worse in 93% of migraine sufferers who also experience frequent auras. It has been demonstrated that surgical closure of the patent foramen ovale reduces the number of migraine days with aura but not the overall number of migraine days when used as a preventive medication.

Despite the fact that treatment responses in migraine with aura are significantly lower than in migraine without aura, the recommended remedies for both types of migraine are the same.

Triptans, the first-line acute treatment for migraine, were found in clinical trials to be ineffective when given during the prodromal stage, when aura typically appears. Sumatriptan injections decreased the average duration of an aura from 30 to 25 minutes, although this marginal reduction was not significantly different from placebo.

Two more recent preventative medications, memantine and lamotrigine, have demonstrated benefit against migraines with and without aura. Due to its various mechanisms of action, topiramate has shown remarkable promise in reducing the frequency of both migraines with and without aura. Only migraines with aura have been linked to a benefit with tonabersat.

Now that a number of major differences between migraines with and without aura are being studied, there is more proof to support their classification as separate diseases. The development of novel therapies for the prevention of migraines with aura may result from further research into the variations in pathophysiologic pathways.

Recurrent headaches known as migraines are characterized by throbbing pain in a particular location of the head. Auras, or warning symptoms, can occasionally occur before migraine attacks. The aura of a migraine headache is absent in a migraine without aura.

Auras or not, migraines, which can last for a few hours to many days, can make it very difficult to do daily tasks. Students with migraines may miss class and suffer in their studies due to headaches.

Although migraines have no established origin, it is thought that they are connected to anomalies in the brain. Since migraines frequently run in families, it is possible that genes are involved. Numerous things, including as exhaustion and lack of sleep, stress, insufficient calorie intake, and hormonal changes, can cause a migraine.

Medication for treating migraines can be obtained from a doctor. Drinking fluids while lying down in a quiet, dark environment can be really helpful.

Migraines are common. The majority of them are treatable with medication and lifestyle changes, despite the fact that they can be incapacitating and force teens to miss school and activities. The best way to treat migraines is to stay away from their causes whenever possible. Almost everyone gets headaches. Many children occasionally have headaches.

How does one tell if a headache is only a passing pain or indicative of anything more serious?

Migraine headaches

Anyone who has ever had a migraine knows how debilitating the pain and accompanying symptoms can be. Read up about what triggers migraines, how they can be treated, and what you can do to avoid getting them in the first place.

• CNS (central nervous system)

Human behavior is controlled by the brain, which has been likened to the supercomputer at the heart of a vast, intricate, and incredibly fast-moving communication network.

Discomfort in the head

Migraine without aura (mo) and migraine with aura (mw) are the two most common migraine subtypes seen in clinical practice (ma). Each subtype has its own distinct set of clinical manifestations and molecular biology risk factors. Migraine headaches typically follow a premonitory phase characterized by neurological symptoms, often involving the eyes or the senses. Migraine manifests in a variety of additional manifestations than these two main categories, such as vestibular, ocular, and/or abdominal migraine. Based on how often episodes occur, migraine can be further characterized as chronic or episodic.

Migraine headaches affect around 38 million people in the United States. They have the sensation of pulsing or throbbing, typically on one side of the brain. Furthermore, they can cause headaches, dizziness, and sensitivity to light and sound. And they can be significantly more painful than the average headache.

However, not every migraine is the same. It's possible that someone else's will differ greatly from yours.

In most cases, "aura" takes the form of a visual phenomenon, such as a series of lines, a shape, or a brief flash. Loss of sight could last anywhere from ten to thirty minutes. Another symptom is a tingling sensation in the limbs. Smell, flavour, touch, and even words can all be affected by an aura's presence.

About 25% of those who get migraines also get an aura. It usually starts an hour or so before a headache hits, and it can linger for as long as the headache itself.

Migraine is also classified into different subgroups.

Seeing auras in the brain stem

Basilar migraine was the previous name for this condition. Slurred speech, vertigo, tinnitus, double vision, unsteadiness, and an acute sensitivity to sound are all part of this, along with other visual, sensory, and speech or language issues.

Migraines that originate in the basilar sinus are unusual. It is possible that your doctor will label your condition "migraine with brain stem aura" to indicate that your headaches originate there.

A person's ability to speak or hear may be impaired, and they may see lines, flashes of light, or spots in their field of vision as a result of this aura. Pain on one or both sides of the head is another symptom that may appear before or with these alterations.

Aura symptoms might last anywhere from two minutes to more than one hour. Depending on the individual, the headache phase may last anywhere from a few hours to multiple days.

Those who have suffered from basilar migraine attacks know how exhausting they can be afterward.

Symptoms

Headaches that originate in the basilar artery Auras from this type of migraine may be similar to those from other types of migraines. In some cases, a person might

- Affect your eyesight in different ways
- Observing zigzag or steady light patterns
- Look for pinpoints or stars
- Have an extreme aversion to loud noises or bright lights
- Feel numb all over, including your face, head, and hands.

Basilar migraine has its own special set of symptoms. Consistent with dependable sources, these include:

- Challenges in Expressing Oneself
- Vertigo
- Tinnitus
- A decline in auditory perception
- Mirror images
- Subpar Muscular Control
- A lowered state of consciousness
- Pain and tingling on both sides of the body
- Anxiety

- Hyperventilation

The onset of moderate to severe pain is often preceded by the onset of aura symptoms. It's possible that the pain in your head will start in one spot and expand from there.

Allodynia may also be brought on by migraine headaches. Light touch, such clothing rubbing against the skin, might be perceived as painful by those who suffer from allodynia.

Migraine symptoms can be different from person to person and from one attack to the next.

Complications

Basilar migraines are characterized by transient sensory disturbances. However, having this type of migraine can increase your risk of developing other health issues, such as an ischemic stroke.

The medical community has several gaps in its understanding of how migraine with aura is linked to an increased risk of stroke.

Combination contraceptive medications may increase the risk of ischemic stroke in women having migraine with aura. Therefore, the WHO does not advise people with this type of migraine to take prescription birth control containing moderate to high amounts of oestrogen.

Stroke risk is also increased by smoking. A person who suffers from basilar migraine could decide to cut down on or give up smoking as a result.

Causes

Basilar migraine, commonly known as migraine with brain stem aura, has no known cause. However, these episodes might be triggered by a variety of environmental factors.

Some of the causes include:

- Stress
- Alcohol

- Caffeine
- The use of nitrites in food
- Constant appetite loss
- Brilliant illumination
- Feeling ill on the road
- Failure to Sleep
- Harsh odors, including some perfumes
- Sudden changes in atmospheric pressure or other weather conditions
- A burdensome load to bear
- Abuse of pain relievers
- Birth control tablets containing hormones
- Hormonal Shifts in Women
- Interventions for Hypertension
- Seizures or epilepsy

Diagnosis

Basilar migraine is usually diagnosed after two or more episodes that meet specific criteria.

Credible origin.

Basilar migraine can look like hemiplegic migraine however the difference is that hemiplegic migraine causes weakness on one side of the body.

Basilar migraine symptoms are similar to those of other, more serious conditions, including as

- Seizures
- Irreversible brain damage
- Meningitis
- Paralysis caused by a stroke

An MRI or CT scan may be ordered by a doctor or neurologist to rule out such conditions.

Treatment

Treatment for basilar migraine often consists of symptom control and pain reduction.

A doctor might suggest:

- ➢ Ibuprofen is one type of the nonsteroidal anti-inflammatory drugs (NSAIDs).
- ➢ Medicines used to prevent or treat vomiting and nausea
- ➢ If OTC remedies aren't doing the trick, your doctor may suggest anything stronger. It's possible you'll be prescribed a medication called a nerve block to help with the pain.

If you experience basilar migraine attacks, it's important to take precautions as soon as you notice the warning signs. Aura symptoms manifest before pain does in most cases. When used before the onset of acute pain, some pain relievers and anti-inflammatory medications tend to be more effective.

Reducing the likelihood of a basilar migraine attack:

Preventative measures, which a doctor may recommend, include:

- ➤ Botox injections
- ➤ Topiramate and other seizure-controlling medications (topamax)
- ➤ Verapamil (Isoptin) is a medication that helps lower blood pressure.

One's ability to reduce the frequency of migraine attacks may also be affected by changes in one's lifestyle. An individual might gain from:

- ✓ Not consuming alcohol or caffeine, which might act as triggers.
- ✓ Maintenance of a regular exercise programme
- ✓ Finding ways to relax and unwind
- ✓ Eating a balanced, nutritious diet
- ✓ Maintenance of a regular sleep schedule
- ✓ Avoiding food insufficiency by eating regularly
- ✓ Limiting Your Exposure to Noise

In addition, these things might help a migraine sufferer:

- Practices that can be implemented in daily life (like yoga)
- Acupuncture
- Behavior modification techniques that focus on the mind and behaviour

When experiencing symptoms, such as those of an aura, it may be best to rest in a dark, quiet place until the symptoms subside. In this situation, pain medication may help even if the patient has not yet experienced any discomfort. Compared to other types of migraines, basilar migraines may be the most debilitating and difficult to treat. However, scientists say that as people age, the frequency and irregularity of the incidents decrease.

A doctor should be consulted by anyone suffering aura symptoms so that other, more severe conditions can be ruled out. Also, if you lose consciousness during a migraine attack, you need to get medical help immediately.

Episodic

If you suffer from migraines, you probably experienced this pattern. It means that you get migraines rarely, perhaps from once a month to seven times a month. A more severe form of migraine, high-frequency episodic migraine or chronic migraine, may be present if you experience headaches or migraine attacks more than seven times per month.

More than a billion people worldwide suffer from migraine, which is a neurological disorder. Migraines are chronic conditions that usually affect a person for several years. You will probably have periodic migraines for the rest of your life.

People with this condition often experience debilitating pain that makes it difficult to go about their regular lives.

You may progress or regress from one migraine symptom to the next, including from episodic to chronic headaches. Migraines occur more frequently in women. Their hormones are always shifting, which may explain this.

Researchers are trying to develop a way to prevent migraines from becoming chronic, as these headaches are much more severe and difficult to treat than their episodic counterparts.

What distinguishes an episodic migraine from a common headache?

People frequently mistake a migraine for a severe headache, but this is not the case. Typically, headaches have no accompanying symptoms. Migraine is a neurological illness with a variety of incapacitating symptoms, including severe headaches.

When you get a migraine, the blood flow in your brain and the surrounding tissue are affected. Throughout an episodic migraine, your brain activity fluctuates.

A migraine may result in a severe headache, however this is not always the case. According to the American migraine prevalence and prevention study, only 42.3% of episodic migraine patients experienced a severe headache.

With episodic migraine, you may suffer additional symptoms in addition to headaches. There are four phases of a migraine, however not everyone suffers all four.

These are some of the most prevalent migraine symptoms:

- Nausea
- Dizziness
- Extreme fatigue
- Heightened perception of light, scent, or sound

Headache is a frequent ailment that can range in intensity from moderate to severe.

If you suffer from migraines frequently, how often do you get migraines versus episodic headaches?

Around 37 million people in the United States suffer from migraines. The distinctions between the two types of migraines are still developing as scientists

The number of migraine days in a month is used by doctors to diagnose episodic migraines. If your monthly migraine frequency ranges from 0 to 14, your condition is considered episodic.

Migraines can be episodic, meaning they come and go, or chronic, meaning they persist constantly. Chronic migraines are much more debilitating and have far-reaching consequences for daily life, and they are a possible progression from episodic migraines. Scientists are looking for a drug that will stop migraines from turning into chronic headaches.

Chronic migraines are much more debilitating, and they raise the likelihood that you'll have secondary medical issues or neurological abnormalities. Migraine headaches occurring on at least 15 days per month for at least three months, with migraine symptoms present on at least 8 of those headache days, is considered chronic migraine.

Persistent migraines may occur less frequently under certain conditions. It is possible to revert back to having episodic headaches if you are experiencing migraine symptoms for fewer than 15 days per month.

Do the same things set off a migraine whether it's a one-time occurrence or a constant problem?

Many people who suffer from migraines try to avoid anything that may trigger their condition because migraine triggers can vary greatly from person to person. In this context, everything that sets off a migraine is called a trigger.

A few common reasons are:

- Anxiety
- Hormonal Shifts in Women
- A lot of noise
- Strenuous exercise routines

- Certain odurs
- Medication
- Problems falling asleep
- Sparkling illuminations
- Weather can be unpredictable.
- Smoking
- Caffeine
- Not eating enough
- Stress

Furthermore, some people's migraines can be triggered by eating particular foods. Examples of frequent offenders are:

- Cheeses with a longer ageing time
- Alcohol
- Chocolate
- Fermented Foods
- Glutamate monosodium (msg)
- Tinned or preserved beef
- Yeast

Many doctors advise keeping a diary to help pinpoint the causes of your migraines. Take notes and keep track of triggers as soon as you notice migraine symptoms. If you keep a journal for a while, you'll be able to go back and identify the situations that set you off and learn to avoid them. In certain cases, this may lessen the severity and frequency of migraine headaches.

Migraine triggers that occur only occasionally:

Although researchers have not pinpointed a single cause for episodic migraines, they have found a variety of risk factors that increase patients' vulnerability to developing the condition. There are currently 37 million Americans, both adults and children, who suffer from migraines. Migraine triggers are out of your control, but being aware of them can help.

You may be more prone to migraines if you do any of the following:

- The sexual identity you were born into.
- Family tree

- Diseases not covered by the NIH
- Migraine headaches are three times more common in people with a female assigned at birth. Hormonal shifts are a known migraine trigger, so it's not surprising that many people experience migraines at specific times of the month.
- Migraine disorders appear to have a genetic component as well. You're more likely to develop migraines if someone in your family has them.
- Migraines are more common in people who already have a medical condition that increases that risk. Anxiety, sadness, sleep disturbances, epilepsy, and bipolar illness all fall under this heading. Most people who suffer from migraines on an episodic basis do not have any underlying medical conditions that would explain their condition.

Is it possible to develop chronic migraine from episodic migraine?

Studies show that 2.5% of individuals who first suffer from episodic migraine go on to experience chronic migraine. Although the causes remain unknown, your likelihood can be predicted using two categories of risk factors. Examples of this are:

- o Risk Factors That Can Be Changed
- o Not easily modified

Among the risk factors that cannot be changed are those such as:

- How old are you?
- Being born into a female gender
- Being less well-educated or less well-respected
- Being so pale
- A person who has suffered a traumatic brain injury

In contrast, addressing risk factors such as these can reduce the likelihood of having chronic migraines.

- Obesity
- Drug Abuse

With the guidance of a doctor, you can make positive changes to your way of life. Effectively lowering the possibility that your migraines may become chronic is a direct result of this.

Diagnose migraine headaches

Migraines cannot be diagnosed with any certainty. Instead, your doctor will focus on symptoms, potential dangers, and previous health. Describe the severity of your migraines, how long they persist, and how frequently they occur.

The examination will involve ruling out other probable explanations of your symptoms since there is no definitive test for detecting episodic migraines. Your doctor may order a variety of diagnostic tests, including a physical examination, bloodwork, and imaging (CT or MRI). This way, they'll know for sure that you have migraines and can help you avoid more attacks.

Methods for Treating Occasional Migraines

Though there is currently no cure for episodic migraines, there are several options for coping with the problem. They have a number of options to choose from depending on the frequency and severity of your migraine attacks, as well as whether or not you suffer from chronic migraines. The multifaceted nature of many diseases necessitates the use of various methods and drugs in tandem.

Treating patients before they get sick

Preventative medications are prescribed by doctors to lessen the occurrence, duration, and intensity of migraine headaches. There's a wide range of options, but these are some of the most common prescriptions from doctors:

- Methysergide
- It's the botulinum toxin, silly.

- Calcium channel blockers (a type of high blood pressure medication)
- Beta-blockers
- Antidepressants
- Prescription drugs that prevent seizures
- Gabapentin, Valproic acid, etc.
- Antibodies that target the calcitonin gene-related peptide (cgrp)
- The anti-epileptic drug topiramate (topamax)

Migraine attacks can be lessened by using certain substances. Some of the most common nutritional supplements are:

• B2

• Magnesium

•Coenzyme

Please with your doctor before beginning any treatment, natural or otherwise.

Termination of pregnancy

If you go to a doctor at the first sign of an episode, they will give you medication to stop it. The goal is to halt the progression of the symptoms into a full-blown assault. Abortion medication can also alleviate some of the distress and sickness that may accompany the procedure.

Many medical professionals recommend using pain relievers such acetaminophen, aspirin, or ibuprofen at the first sign of a migraine. They may also prescribe the following drugs to help you feel better:

Mediciness that prevent nausea and vomiting

- It's the botulinum toxin, silly.
- Calcitonin antagonists; peptides that block the effects of the calcitonin gene (cgrp)
- Ditans
- Dopamine receptor blockers
- Ergotamines
- Gepants
- Triptans
- Emergency care

Rescue medicine is typically prescribed for 7-10 days when an abortion therapy fails. Although they can not stop migraines from happening, some medications can help ease their effects.

- Medicines in this category include:
- Medications to prevent sickness
- Medication to prevent seizures
- Dihydroergotamine, to be specific (dhe)
- Relaxants for tense muscles
- Strong anaesthetic pain relievers
- Steroids

Your doctor may recommend intravenous medication for severe cases that have not responded to other treatments.

Healing with a holistic approach:

The medical community strongly supports patients having access to a variety of treatment alternatives. Migraine attacks can be avoided, and their severity can be lessened or even eliminated, with their help. In order to determine which medications would be best suited to your needs, it is recommended that you speak with your primary care physician.

When will a doctor advise against treating migraines if they only occur occasionally?

Preventive treatment could help about 38% of people who suffer from episodic migraines (prophylaxis). The actual percentage of people who use these medications is significantly lower than 13%. Talk to your doctor about how you're feeling right now to see whether preventative measures are necessary.

Your doctor will decide if preventative migraine treatment is necessary after considering the severity and frequency of your headaches. Your doctor is more likely to prescribe preventative medication if you have four or more episodes per month3, especially if your symptoms are severe and linger for at least eight days each time.

Migraine preventative drugs may have the following side effects and risks:

Preventative medications are generally well tolerated, yet the risk for harm with any given medication must always be considered. Migraines can be so debilitating that in many cases, taking the chance of finding relief is warranted. Before deciding on a treatment plan, it's important to sit down with your doctor and talk about the benefits and drawbacks of each option.

To give just one example, amitriptyline has been shown to have the most severe potential for adverse effects. Some of the most common are:

- Sedation
- Confused perception
- Constipation
- Lack of saliva production
- Abnormal heartbeats
- Tachycardia
- Incidence of retentive urinary incontinence

- Diseases of the heart's electrical system
- Orthostatic Hypotension
- Prolonged Qt interval
- Putting on Weight

The following are possible negative effects of other preventative medications:

- Nausea
- Tremors
- Birth Defects In The Nervous System, Also Known As Neural Tube Defect (if pregnant)
- Weakness in the Stomach
- Issues with recall
- Concentration issues
- A stone in the kidney
- Weight reduction
- The Changing Palate

If you think preventative care is warranted in your case, bring it up with your doctor. You two can weigh the potential for harmful repercussions against the potential benefits.

When should I see a doctor?

Less than half of those who experience migraines currently seek medical help. Consequently, fewer than half of people who experience migraines get the care they need to recover.

Finding out if your migraines are under control is crucial. If you have symptoms more than once a week, or if you haven't found a prescription that helps, it's time to see a doctor. They can help you come up with a strategy to deal with your migraines.

Many people in the United States, both young and old, suffer from migraines, which is a neurological disorder. Studies show that one billion people around the world endure the agony of migraine headaches. Among the symptoms include headaches ranging from mild to severe, nausea, dizziness, tiredness, and sensitivity to bright lights, odours, and sounds.

While migraines cannot be cured, there are several treatments available to help patients cope with the pain and avoid further episodes. Make an appointment with your doctor if your episodic migraines are affecting your everyday life and medication isn't helping. Your treatment plan to reduce your migraine attacks will be developed by these professionals.

Occurring frequently:

This type of migraine is characterized by having between eight and fourteen days of headaches per month. The risk of having chronic migraine is also raised.

Chapter 3

Four phases of an intermittent migraine

A migraine episode can be divided into four segments. It is not always the case that each phase is accompanied by distinct symptoms. Some individuals have all four phases with several symptoms, while others experience only one or two. Consider the four phases of the episodic migraine.

Prodromal period

The prodromal phase, also known as the pre-headache phase, indicates the onset of a migraine attack. This phase's symptoms are typically painless and might occur hours to days prior to the onset of a migraine.

During the prodromal period, you might experience the following:

- Nausea
- Irritability
- Increased urine output
- Fatigue
- Depression
- Having trouble sleeping
- Difficulty focusing, reading, or communicating
- Extreme yawning
- Food desires
- Light, odors, or sound sensitivity
- Rigid muscles

Aura phase

During the aura phase, you may feel alterations to your hearing, vision, and/or speech. An aura is not usually present before a migraine headache, but experiencing one for the first time might be unsettling. Symptoms of aura phase:

- Visual impairments such as impaired vision
- Blind patches
- And zigzag patterns

> ➢ Tingling or numbness in the arms, legs, or face
> ➢ Problems with speech such as slurring or jumbling words
> ➢ Experience visual disturbances

Many individuals with episodic migraines learn to recognize an aura so they can prepare for the subsequent phase before it begins. Preparation may involve taking pain medication or cancelling plans in order to be at home.

Headache period

Some migraine sufferers do not have a headache during the headache phase. Headache pain can range from mild to severe. Certain physical activities and sensations can exacerbate pain, thus many individuals attempt to avoid certain pungent odors, loud noises, and bright lights.

When having an episodic migraine, the headache is frequently described as throbbing, stabbing, or pounding.

Additionally, some individuals remark that it feels like great pressure.

In addition to headaches, the headache phase might cause you to feel:

> Nausea (with or without vomiting)
> Dizziness
> Congestion
> Anxious
> Unable to sleep
> Irritable
> Sensitive to light, smell, or sound
> Tired
> Pain and stiffness in their neck

Postdrome phase

Once the headache goes away, the postdrome phase begins. This can generate different symptoms and emotions, most of which are not pleasant. Some of the most prevalent feelings include:

- Confusion
- Exhaustion
- Feeling ill

Chapter 4

SEX,GENDER AND MIGRAINE

In this chapter, we will discuss the sex and gender dynamics that contribute to the prevalence of epidemic headaches.

- Women are more likely to get migraines, and they tend to be more severe, frequent, and debilitating. Migraine symptoms and accompanying conditions might vary greatly from person to person. Women, in particular, are predisposed to experiencing migraine symptoms such nausea, photophobia, and phonophobia. Sex hormones, like oestrogen, play a role in migraine pathogenesis. Oestrogen withdrawal is a known migraine trigger. Other hormones, such as progesterone and testosterone, are less well understood. In both human and animal studies, researchers have found links between cgrp (the target of novel acute and preventative migraine medications) and sex hormones. Migraines are linked to puberty, pregnancy, and menopause/postmenopause, as shown by their natural lifecycle progression. In the case of menstrual migraine, the usage of hormone-containing therapies is still up for debate. The risk of stroke appears to vary with both oestrogen dose and aura frequency, according to a reanalysis of the available data. There are hardly any data on the prevalence of migraines among people of non-binary genders. Hormone therapy to achieve a desired gender has the potential to alter migraines and other symptoms associated with menstrual imbalance (including ischemic stroke with high dose estrogen).

- Sex hormones are thought to play a role in migraine pathogenesis and the natural progression of migraine over the course of a person's lifetime, both of which contribute to important disparities in migraine epidemiology and symptomatology. Therapies for menstrual migraine that are more specific and effective are needed. A comprehensive review of the literature on oestrogen and stroke risk suggests that a nuanced strategy toward the use of contraception and hormone replacement therapy containing oestrogen is required. Limited but expanding research on the link between gender affirming therapy and migraine, as well as treatment concerns for transgender individuals with migraine, contribute to our growing knowledge of sex and gender.

Perspectives on sex, gender, and migraine attack

- Throughout history, there has been a gradual expansion of both the social and scientific consensus on how we should conceptualise sex and gender. In the 1950s, psychologist john money and his colleagues initially distinguished between sex and gender, holding that the former reflected physical qualities while the latter were determined by one's actions and mindset [1, 2, 3]. For the purpose of this article, we shall use the widely accepted definitions from the American Psychological Association's (APA) standards on sexual orientation and gender diversity, despite the fact that there is some room for interpretation in these areas.

- The term "sex" is used to describe a person's biological gender, which might be male, female, or intersex. External and internal genitalia, as well as sex chromosomes, are used as indications of biological sex.
- The term "gender" is used to describe the socially constructed associations between a person's psychological and behavioural states and their biological sex.

- Medical studies typically blur the lines between sex as a biological reality and gender as a social construction. This haziness has important ramifications for our knowledge of migraine prevalence and aetiology, particularly in groups that are not homogenous by sex. Most studies only collect information about sex or gender in a binary format (such as female/male or woman/man) and do not distinguish between biological sex and gender expression. The physical traits of a newborn are used to determine the sex assigned at birth (saab). On the other side, a person's gender identity is not dependent on their saab (though it often coincides with it) and describes their subjective experiences of being male, female, or ambiguous. The outward manifestation of a person's gender in their behaviour, clothing, voice, etc. is what is meant by "gender expression," which is different from "gender identity." Each and every person has their own unique combination of these characteristics. Sexual orientation, which is defined as a person's romantic, sexual, or emotional attraction to others, is not a factor in any of these aspects of identity. The majority of studies on migraines fail to distinguish between saab and gender identity, and even less evaluate sexual orientation and gender expression. This perspective limits our ability to ascertain whether gender-based differences in migraine prevalence result from biological differences, hormonal distinctions, or differing exposure to the psychosocial pressures associated with gender identity and expression.

- This way of thinking also limits our ability to comprehend migraine in gm communities. People whose gender identity or expression does not conform to saab norms are collectively referred to as "gm," an umbrella word that encompasses all such people. That includes, but is not limited to, people who identify as transgender, gender non-conforming, or who don't identify with either gender. Migraine research in the gm community is hampered by the lack of large, well-controlled studies and the substantial risk of bias inherent in observational research because of the lack of information about gender identity outside of saab.

- Unfortunately, the vast majority of the cited studies treat gender and sex as interchangeable, and their study methods may not make it clear which was examined. Unless otherwise specified, references to women and men in this article will be to cisgender (non-transgender) women and men. We will explore migraine epidemiology, co-morbid illnesses, and symptomatology in connection to gender and sexual orientation. We will also talk about how sex hormones play a role in migraine pathogenesis and how patients can benefit from treatments that include hormones. Throughout, we will highlight discoveries related to gm as well as briefly discuss gender affirming hormone therapy and special migraine concerns in transgender individuals.

Epidemiology

- Women are two to three times more likely to experience migraines than men do, both in the US and internationally. In addition to having a higher incidence of migraine, women also had a higher prevalence of headache-related disability, used more prescription and over-the-counter medications to treat their headaches, and were more likely to take prescription medications to treat their depression or anxiety. There was also an increase in visits to urgent care clinics and emergency rooms. While more women than ever before are entering the workforce, it is still mostly women (even those who work full time) who are responsible for the majority of housework. Migraine during menstruation, which can be more severe and, as a result, more debilitating, is another issue. The research study found some intriguing trends in men, such as the lower prevalence of migraine diagnoses in men and the higher prevalence of co-morbid cardiac illness and stroke, emphysema, and hypertension compared to allergies, asthma, temporomandibular disorders, anxiety, and raynaud's in women. Men experienced fewer attacks, less allodynia, and fewer aura symptoms overall compared to women. There was a marked increase in the risk of chronic migraine among men with a history of episodic migraine. History of head trauma (more common in men) may play a role in how severe migraines become, however this was not assessed. Additional research is needed to verify these results.

Data collection for the Migraine in America Study of Symptoms and Treatment (mast) began in 2016 with the overarching goal of analysing migraine symptoms, diagnosis, management, and co-morbidities; the study intends to update migraine epidemiologic information. Similar to earlier epidemiological studies, 2018 data on sex differences indicated that women experience more impairment and more frequent headache days than men. It's worth noting that the survey did not capture any data that could be considered inclusive, as respondents were asked to identify as either male or female. Sixty-three percent of the study population displayed headache frequency indicative of episodic migraine (1-4 mhd/mo), whereas less than ten percent exhibited headache frequency indicative of chronic migraine (at least 15 mhd/mo). Women were overrepresented in the groups with chronic migraine and high-frequency episodic migraine (10-14 mhd).

Prospective online enrollment for the Observational Survey of Migraine Epidemiology, Treatment, and Care (Overcome) Research began in 2018. Up to this point, data from a sample of over 20,000 people who met criteria for migraines in the spring of 2019 showed a correlation between high-quality acute therapy for migraines and fewer migraine-related disability days and better health-related quality of life. The study's design prevented collecting data from members of gender minorities, and the results that were broken down by sex and gender have yet to be published.

The migraine epidemic among gm communities is poorly understood. Six headache-related papers (four case reports and two cross-sectional studies) were found by a 2021 scoping analysis of sgm literature in neurology. Only the cross-sectional study looked at migraine, and only one of those studies even included transgender people.

Comorbidities in Migraine

An individual's comorbidity describes an association between two conditions that is not due to chance alone. Identifying comorbidities in migraine patients may help researchers better understand the disease's pathophysiology, develop more effective treatments, and identify previously unknown risk factors. Recent epidemiological data from mast research indicates that sleep disturbance, depression, anxiety, and gastric ulcer/gi haemorrhage are the most common comorbid conditions. The chance of having many mental health conditions is affected by social and demographic factors. The prevalence of co-morbid anxiety was shown to be lower among married, employed, male, and older adults (65+). Depression is also less common in those who are older, who have families, who are gainfully employed, and who have a higher standard of living. The prevalence of mhd was positively correlated with the presence of mental and nonpsychiatric comorbidities. Comorbidities in gm migraine patients cannot be assessed at this time because to a lack of data.

The Signs of a Migraine Attack

- Migraine is defined by the current ichd-3 as a headache that is unilateral in site, quality (pulsating or throbbing), severity (moderate or severe), duration (greater than four hours), and comorbid symptoms (nausea and/or vomiting, photophobia, and phonophobia). Some people with migraines experience more nausea or photophobia than pain, while others experience the opposite. Migraine symptoms like nausea, sensitivity to light and sound, and a heightened sensitivity to sound were found to be more common in females, and migraine attacks lasted longer and were more severe, according to one of the earliest studies to examine the impact of gender on migraine symptoms. In contrast to men, symptomatology in women changed with age. Although the term gender is used throughout the research, it is not made clear whether or not the researchers focused on sex or gender according to apa norms. Similar gender differences can be seen in the ampp data. Migraine headaches affected the majority of those who responded (1–4 mhds). Pain levels were almost the same between the sexes on average, however migraines were more commonly diagnosed in women (nausea, vomiting, photophobia, phonophobia, visual aura). In terms of function, women were more likely to report needing bed rest and experiencing a longer duration of impairment compared to males, who reported being able to continue functioning and experiencing a shorter time of post-migraine impairment.

Substances with a role in pathophysiology

It is widely thought that sex hormones play a role in the observed epidemiological differences in migraine prevalence by sex, although the underlying processes behind this pattern remain poorly understood. Over the past few decades, our understanding of the mechanisms producing migraine has expanded, revealing a complex interplay between events such as vascular changes, hyperexcitability, neurotransmitter and neuropeptide signalling, and activation of functional brain networks. This article discusses the role of sexual hormones in the aetiology and pathophysiology of migraines.

The causes of migraines

A premonitory period of hypothalamic, brainstem, and cortical activity precedes migraine attacks and is associated with changes in mood, fatigue, food cravings, yawning, neck pain, or sensitivity to stimuli (light, sound). Aura is characterised by reversible neurologic symptoms (most usually visual) that manifest before the onset of headache pain and are thought to be caused by cortical spreading depolarization (a wave of neuronal depolarization). It's also possible to have an aura before or alongside a headache. Pain in the head is felt when the trigeminal vascular system is stimulated. A functional pathway, the trigeminovascular system relays nociception from the meninges and cerebral arteries to the trigeminocervical complex (tcc) (composed of the trigeminal nucleus caudalis and the upper cervical dorsal horn) in the brainstem, and from there to the hypothalamus, thalamus, and cortical regions. Pain in various regions of the face, head, and neck is caused by the convergence of sensory and nociceptive inputs from the trigeminal ganglion and other trigeminal and cervical structures. Cortical processing of pain signals is likely the underlying cause of migraine symptoms like sensitivity to stimuli and cognitive impairments. Calcitonin gene-related peptide (cgrp), substance p, and pituitary adenosine cyclase-activating polypeptide-38 are all secreted into the perivascular space by dural nociceptive afferents in response to activation of the trigeminovascular system. This leads to a phenomenon called neurogenic vasodilation. The trigeminal ganglion and the trigeminal cochlear nucleus are two further areas where Cgrp is active (tcc). In the case of trigeminovascular neuronal sensitization, the threshold for responses is lowered while the magnitude of responses to dural stimulation is amplified. This mechanism may account for the throbbing quality and movement-induced aggravation of migraine pain. It's possible that Cgrp and other factors contribute. Central sensitization, manifested clinically as cephalic and extracephalic cutaneous allodynia, may result from chronic trigeminovascular activation.

Stress and migraines

During the late luteal (premenstrual) phase of the menstrual cycle, oestrogen levels drop, which is linked to an increase in migraine headaches. A recent study of sex hormone levels found that migraine sufferers had a faster decline in oestrogen levels during the luteal phase than controls; however, this decline was not always accompanied by a migraine attack, suggesting that it is a susceptibility factor that may facilitate migraine if triggered by other factors (change in sleep, stress, or other individual triggers). Women who had migraines before menopause were the only ones for whom a decline in exogenously supplied oestrogen was associated with migraine onset, suggesting an innate susceptibility to hormonal changes in migraine sufferers. Estradiol levels were found to be significantly higher in non-obese guys with migraine, according to a recent study (as well as clinical evidence of androgen deficit). Oestrogen has been shown to increase sensitivity to cortical spreading depolarization and responses from the trigeminovascular system in animal studies. Migraines with aura are more common in women who are pregnant or who use hormonal contraception or hormone replacement therapy.

Although oestrogen has received the most attention, other hormones, such as progesterone and testosterone, may also play a role in migraines. Circulating hormones (such as oestrogen, progesterone, and testosterone) can enter the brain because they are lipophilic molecules. Their primary function is to act as building blocks in the nervous system, where they eventually get converted into neurosteroids. Since allopregnanolone (a progesterone and pregnenolone derivative) is the centrally active progesterone in the cns, and since it inhibits neuronal excitability by enhancing gaba activity, this mechanism is important for progesterone (as a gaba receptor modulator). It is thought that progesterone withdrawal explains catamenial epilepsy because it lowers the seizure threshold in animal models of epilepsy. Like in epilepsy, migraine can be caused by an overactive cortex. Progesterone is thought to have a neuroprotective effect by reducing nociception in the trigeminovascular system. Despite similar serum progesterone levels between those with migraine and controls, a recently published cross-sectional pilot study found that serum allopregnanolone levels in women with migraine were lower, and this was inversely related to migraine duration and frequency. This observation may be associated with the neuroprotective effects of allopregnanolone, which may reduce neurogenic inflammation in migraine patients (that can, in turn, contribute to central sensitization and chronification).

However, the role of testosterone in migraines is poorly understood. Subcutaneous testosterone implants reduced headache severity in a prospective pilot study of women (pre- and post-menopausal) with migraine (episodic vs. chronic, not specified). Importantly, there are major limitations to this study, including the fact that the patient population had androgen deficiency symptoms, there was no control group (degree of placebo effect unknown), and the outcome was an assessment of headache intensity (5-point scale) rather than interval assessment of headache frequency (mhds) or use of a validated instrument to measure change after a therapeutic intervention (hit-6, midas). Danazol (an androgen) was used in a small study, and the results showed a decrease in "hormonal migraine" (menstrual migraine). Men with chronic migraine have lower testosterone levels compared to controls, according to recent prospective observational pilot research. Testosterone may reduce the severity of migraines by lowering cortical spreading depolarization, increasing serotonin, maintaining cerebral blood flow, and exhibiting neuroprotective and anti-inflammatory properties. High rates of migraine with aura were found in the Dutch study of transgender women taking hormone therapy (antiandrogens and estrogens), which is in line with what has been seen in cisgender women taking oestrogen replacement therapy.

Hormonal and cgrp

As cgrp-targeting acute and preventative treatments for migraines have become more widely available, the connections between cgrp and sex hormones have been investigated in animal models. Recent studies have shown that oestrogen receptors can influence cgrp production and receptor signalling in the trigeminovascular system, and that these effects are influenced by cyclical fluctuations in oestrogen levels. Experimental evidence from animals suggests that the excitability and sensitization of the cgrp pathway is influenced by estrogens, and that cgrp system activation varies with the estrous cycle. Estradiol induced oestrogen receptor-mediated neurogenic vasodilation and spread depolarization in rat cortices. This sensitivity is enhanced in healthy females when oestrogen levels are low, as shown by an experimental model of crgrp release from sensory neurons in the dermis in response to capsaicin. Migraine sufferers' responses were more intense than those of non-migraine sufferers', but they did not change over the course of a woman's menstrual cycle. Consistent with previous research showing a reduction in oestrogen is associated with migraine risk, this shows a higher cgrp response in migraine sufferers and an influence of oestrogen on cgrp. In addition to cyclical changes in oestrogen, the onset of menstruation is accompanied by a rise in prostaglandin levels that trigger the release of neuroinflammatory mediators like substance P, neurokinins, and cgrp. This interplay between hormones and cgrp is reflected in the fact that both pregnancy and menopause—stages characterized by changes in sex hormones—are linked to shifts in circulating cgrp.

Hormonal interactions and the typical progression of migraines

Hormones may play a role in the differences in the onset and prevalence of migraines between genders and different stages of life. For children under the age of puberty, the prevalence over a period of one year is similar for boys and girls between the ages of 9 and 10 (2-5%) and 10 to 12 (4-5%). This trend breaks down around the time of puberty. The prevalence is on the rise among both boys and girls, though the increase among girls is more pronounced (6% versus 4%). There is no decrease in the lifetime prevalence of migraine in women. Both men and women experience a peak in migraine prevalence between the ages of 35 and 50, and then a gradual decline thereafter; however, the natural course of migraines tends to be more consistent in men. Hormonal influence is further suggested by the fact that at least 20% of women with migraine also experience menstrually associated migraine and that migraine symptoms change (usually for the better) during pregnancy and menopause. Women who suffer from menstrual migraine may be more likely to have their headaches subside during pregnancy and then worsen following perimenopause. Researchers believe that shifts in oestrogen and progesterone levels, particularly more frequent and longer episodes of oestrogen withdrawal, play a role in triggering perimenopause. Migraine frequency seems to lessen after menopause.

Migraines are more common and disabling in women, and some statistics suggest that transfeminine people also experience a higher migraine prevalence. To gain a fuller understanding of migraine in gm patients, further epidemiology studies are required. Migraine symptoms and associated conditions appear to differ between the sexes. These differences are often attributed to differences in sex hormones that develop during development. Oestrogen regulates aspects of migraine pathogenesis, such as cortical spreading depolarization, trigeminovascular activation, and cgrp signalling, in both animal and human models. Hormonal changes cause a shift in migraine incidence during adolescence, and women have both mild and severe migraines at different times during pregnancy and menopause.

- **Migraines associated with menstruation**

Until more study and validation can be conducted, the diagnostic criteria for menstrual migraine will remain in the ichd-3 appendix. Migraine attacks that occur only during the perimenstrual period (before and during menstruation) are called "pure menstrual migraine," while "menstrually associated migraine" includes perimenstrual attacks as well as other types of migraine. These definitions are sufficient because of the infrequent occurrence of attacks typical of episodic migraine. A chronic migraine sufferer may, however, experience an attack during the perimenstrual phase, thereby fitting the criteria for menstrually associated migraine. However, different studies may use different criteria to define menstrual migraine, making it hard to draw consistent conclusions about the condition's prevalence or even to make comparisons between studies. Prevalence estimates are also affected by the study population. Estimates of the prevalence of migraine in the general population range from 18-25%, whereas in headache clinics, the prevalence of menstrual migraine (without aura) is 22-70%. In studies reporting a higher prevalence, the criteria for defining menstrual migraine are generally less stringent. Oral contraceptive side effects further complicate matters because headaches are common during the placebo/hormone-free week and may be unique from headaches that occur during non-hormone-influenced menstrual cycles.

Multiple studies have shown that perimenstrual migraine attacks are more severe, disabling, and long-lasting than other types of migraine attacks, and that they are also less responsive to treatment and more likely to be accompanied by symptoms including sensitivity to stimuli and nausea. But there are currently no FDA-approved treatments for migraines that occur during the perimenstrual period. Discovering efficient short-term treatments for those who experience episodic migraines is a top priority. Individuals with episodic migraine and monthly migraine should weigh the frequency, intensity, and overall sickness burden when deciding whether to begin migraine prophylaxis. Short-term perimenstrual prophylaxis should be addressed in addition to acute or preventative therapy. The off-label use of frovatriptan for the avoidance of perimenstrual attacks is common and supported by some data (begun a few days prior to the predicted onset of menstruation and continued during menstruation). Naratriptan and zolmitriptan are two other short-term preventative triptans. The following discussion focuses on the use of hormonal contraceptives in the treatment of menstrual migraines.

HRT and oral contraceptives.

However, there is a dearth of information on the effectiveness of hormonal treatments for migraine, such as oral contraceptives (ocps) and hormone replacement therapy (hrt) in postmenopausal women, despite the pathophysiological link between hormones and migraine. There is some evidence to support the use of continuous, low-dose estrogen-containing contraception, which minimises fluctuations in oestrogen, or regimens that limit the decline in oestrogen (to 10 ug), which triggers migraine, in the event that standard acute and preventive treatments for menstrual migraine continue to be ineffective. Migraine sufferers who also had aura were not included in studies evaluating the efficacy of continuous regimen oral contraceptives for the treatment of menstrual migraines because of the controversy surrounding the use of contraception containing oestrogen. Migraine with aura is related with a twofold greater risk of ischemic stroke, even after adjusting for other risk factors. Oral contraceptives with oestrogen have always been considered a bad idea for people who suffer from migraines with aura (which may increase the risk of stroke). Alternative approaches (progestin-only, intrauterine devices) are preferred if used purely for contraception. This assertion, however, has been challenged by some who have reexamined the evidence and found it wanting. When oestrogen levels were higher (in 1975), the first report of an association between ocps and stroke risk was published (for example, 100–150 ug mestranol, the popular dose for oral contraception in the 1960s-1970s). Stroke risk appears to be dose-dependent, with no correlation seen between the lower risk and lower dosages in recent research. These days, only around 1 in 100 oral contraceptives have the required 50 ug of ethinyl estradiol. Furthermore, both a meta-analysis of many U.S. trials and a large-scale investigation found that low-dose ocps did not increase the risk of stroke. The frequency of auras is a factor in risk assessment alongside oestrogen dose. Ischemic stroke risk increases in proportion to the number of times an aura occurs. Conclusion: Migraine sufferers who have auras should avoid estrogen-containing ocps if at all possible, but a more tailored approach will require data on aura frequency and oestrogen dose. Another option is hormone replacement therapy that does not involve taking pills. Continuous use of a vaginal ring containing a modest dose of ethinyl estradiol (15 ug/24 h) lowered aura frequency and improved menstrual migraine in > 90% of participants in a clinic-based retrospective analysis of individuals with migraine with aura and intractable menstrually-related migraine.

The outcomes of the few studies done on hrt and migraines during menopause were inconsistent. There is a lack of information for women over the age of 50 because most studies assessing the risk of stroke in migraine with aura have been undertaken on younger people. One study looked at the link between hrt and ischemic stroke in women with migraines and found no evidence of one; however, the study lacked important details about the hrt being used (type, dose, and route). Transdermal low-dose oestrogen may reduce the oestrogen swings linked to migraine onset and alleviate the vasomotor symptoms of menopause without significantly increasing the risk of stroke. However, increased risk of new migraines with aura and worsening of existing migraines have also been linked to high doses of oral oestrogen. Hormone replacement medication must be discontinued if an existing migraine worsens or a new migraine with aura develops.

Hormone therapy to affirm gender and the relief of migraines

Migraine frequency and impairment are not adequately studied in relation to gender affirming hormone therapy (gaht). Not all gm people take gaht; the hormones, if any, a person decides to use to achieve their gender affirmation is a personal decision. A single Italian study looked at how gaht affected pain in 47 transgender women and 26 transgender men, with a focus on headache as the pain endpoint. Of the 14 transgender women who complained of ongoing pain, 3 said their headaches started after they started gaht, whereas 2 said theirs started before they started gaht but got worse after they started. The majority of patients (10) reported headaches before starting gaht, with different responses after the introduction of testosterone: improvement in six, no change in three, and worsening in one. Although the specific cause of headaches in transgender people is not determined by this study, it does detail the experiences of transwomen who suffer from this condition, including photophobia and phonophobia, as well as the experiences of transmen who have a family history of headaches. Furthermore, it is unclear if and how gender-affirming surgeries impact the frequency and intensity of migraine attacks.

The gaht-based management of migraine in transgender patients relies heavily on consensus due to a paucity of data. Oestrogen levels should be monitored to make sure they stay within normal physiological parameters, and consistent oestrogen levels are especially critical for transfeminine people to accomplish. Migraines in transmasculinity have been linked to oestrogen variations caused by persistent ovarian activity, even in the absence of menstruation. Intramuscular medroxyprogesterone acetate may help in this situation. Gaht may interact with migraine prophylaxis treatments, especially antiepileptic drugs, thus it's important to be aware of this possibility. Medications used to treat epilepsy, like topiramate and valproic acid, can interfere with the body's metabolism of estrogens, progestins, and testosterone by inhibiting the cyp 3a4 pathway. Although this may have implications for transgender patients' clinical care, the only studies describing this connection are from cisgender populations. Gender affirming therapy that is both lifesaving and medically required. The patient and prescriber of gender affirming care should work together to alter migraine treatment or the formulation/type of gaht if there is concern about a potential interaction.

Transgender people and migraine treatment

Transgender people require specialised medical attention in addition to the standard diagnostic tests and treatments for migraine. Caretakers need to be aware of the risks associated with gaht. Secondary polycythemia, a side effect of masculinizing drugs like testosterone, can cause headaches and increase the likelihood of migraine aura. When it comes to feminising hormones, research suggests that taking larger dosages of oral oestrogen can raise your risk of venous thrombosis, stroke, and cardiovascular disease. Additionally, cyproterone acetate can cause tumours of the prolactin gland and the meninges if taken in excessive amounts. Due to the seriousness of the risks involved, it is essential to be on the lookout for secondary headache triggers. Risk assessment is based on data from the cisgender women's community, but there is a lack of information about the risk of ischemic stroke in transgender women with migraine who use oestrogen therapy.

Providers may also notice an increase in migraine and migraine aura in patients on feminising medicines due to the pathophysiologic effects of oestrogen on the trigeminovascular system and cortical spreading depolarization. There is some indication that transgender males have a lower incidence of migraines, although the effect of testosterone on migraines has not been fully investigated. Preclinical studies suggest that testosterone's anti-nociceptive and anti-inflammatory actions may result from its ability to inhibit the spreading depolarization of neurons in the cortex.

Migraine with aura is associated with an elevated risk of ischemic stroke in transgender patients taking estrogen-containing drugs; therefore, clinicians should encourage patients to minimise cigarette use and manage other vascular risk factors to lower this risk (diabetes, hypertension, and hyperlipidemia).

Issues of health inequality, socioeconomic status, and research bias

Migraine incidence, prevalence, and outcomes are impacted by structural and socioeconomic determinants of health, just as they are for other neurologic disorders. Although a thorough analysis of migraine inequalities is outside the scope of this review, this article will focus on the ways in which sex and gender are just two of many personal and social identities that may affect migraine prevalence and severity. The idea of intersectionality is crucial to this process. Intersectionality is the experience of numerous forms of oppression due to membership in different social minorities. So far as we can tell, there are no intersectional studies of episodic migraine. Previous research has shown that there are significant racial/ethnic, socioeconomic, and sexual orientation gaps in the prevalence of self-reported migraines. Access to effective headache treatment is also affected by socioeconomic and gender-related factors. A 2006 editorial argued that the fact that men are less likely to seek care for headaches and are less likely to be diagnosed with migraines is due in part to pharmaceutical marketing aimed at women, which in turn creates hurdles for headache treatment. In order to broaden these studies and comprehend the impact of new and contemporaneous social determinants of health, more study is required.

Previous justification for using predominantly male animal models of migraine was to reduce the impact of varying sex hormones on outcomes, despite the fact that migraine is more common in women. In contrast, female participants are overrepresented in human clinical trials, restricting extrapolation to the still significant proportion of males who suffer from migraine. National institutes of health funding for the study of sex as a variable in both animal and human studies has expanded, giving new alternatives for future exploration.

Chronic

This headache has been happening at least 15 times a month for over three months. At least eight days a month, you suffer from migraine headaches.

Hemiplegic

This word refers to paralysis that affects only one side of the body. A temporary (less than 72 hours) weakness on one side of the body is caused by the aura that accompanies these headaches. The symptoms of an aura usually subside after 24 hours.

There is no permanent nerve damage, but the symptoms are quite similar to a stroke.

Don't try to play doctor just yet! Seek emergency medical assistance if you experience symptoms consistent with a hemiplegic migraine and make sure a stroke is not the cause.

Subtle Headache

In fact, migraines can happen even if you don't feel any pain in your head. A silent migraine is the most prevalent type of migraine.

The most noticeable precursor to this form of migraine is aura. There are several migraine symptoms, including nausea. Twenty to thirty minutes is a common range.

Chronic abdominal migraine

A type of migraine in which the pain originates in the stomach rather than the brain. Some of the signs include:

- Body Ache
- Nausea
- A decrease in appetite
- Vomiting

Migraines in the abdomen can affect adults. However, they tend to impact young people who themselves experience migraines or who have close relatives who do.

The causes of these conditions are unknown to the medical community. However, they have many of the same causes as regular migraines. And medications for migraines are really good at alleviating the pain.

Menstrual

In most cases, they start two days before a woman's menstruation and end three days following. Migraine headaches can manifest differently for different women at different times of the month, but migraines associated with menstruation are often headaches without aura.

Ocular (or retinal)

Rarely does a person suffer from this kind of migraine. It causes changes in vision, such as perceiving colours where none exist, seeing flashing lights, or going blind in one eye. The migraine headache that follows the temporary blindness is expected to be typical. There are, however, significant conditions that can cause sudden loss of vision in one eye; if you notice any changes in your vision, you should consult a doctor right away.

Vestibular

Vertigo is a common symptom of a migraine of this kind. The duration of this spinning feeling can range from minutes to hours.

Headache condition known as status migrainosus

Status migrainosus is characterised by pain that lasts longer than three days. Certain drugs and the discontinuation of others can trigger it.

This type of migraine can cause severe pain and nausea, potentially necessitating hospitalisation. In this circumstance, it's imperative that you get assistance right away.

Migraine attacks characterised by drooping eyelids

If you're experiencing pain or weakness in the area of your eye, you should consult a doctor right away. It's possible that the cause of these strange symptoms is ophthalmoplegic migraine (today called neuralgia), or it could be something more serious. Ophthalmoplegic migraines can cause double vision, drooping eyelids, and other visual disturbances, and they often endure for a week.

If you're experiencing any of the following, don't hesitate to see a doctor:

• Variation in migraine type, migraine frequency, or migraine intensity.

Symptoms such as:

- A persistent headache that gets worse with time

- A painful and distracting head ache from excessive coughing, sneezing, bending over, or straining at the toilet.

- If you think you need to go to the ER, consider these situations:

- If you've ever had a severe headache that came on abruptly, it qualifies.

- Pain in the head after a blow to the head

- Consciousness loss due to head trauma

- Headache and/or high body temperature

- Disorientation or amnesia

- Weakness or inability to move

- Seizure

- shift in perspective

- Reduced eyesight.

Chapter 5

Theories concerning migraine pain

Historically, it was believed that migraine symptoms were caused by variations in blood flow to the brain. Many headache researchers now recognize that changes in blood flow and blood vessels may not cause headaches, but may contribute to them.

As new technology and research have paved the path for a deeper knowledge, the current understanding of migraine discomfort has shifted to focus on the problem's root cause. Today, it is generally accepted that chemical substances and hormones, such as serotonin and oestrogen, frequently have a role in migraine patients' pain sensitivity.

A component of the hypothesis of migraine pain suggests that migraine pain is caused by waves of brain cell activity. These cause neurotransmitters like serotonin to constrict blood arteries. Serotonin is a neurotransmitter required for nerve cell transmission. It can cause blood vessel constriction throughout the body.

When serotonin or oestrogen levels fluctuate, some people experience migraines. Serotonin levels can impact both sexes, whereas oestrogen levels only effect women.

Estrogen levels fluctuate naturally throughout a woman's life, increasing during her reproductive years and decreasing subsequently. Menstruating women experience monthly fluctuations in oestrogen levels. The correlation between migraines in women and fluctuating hormone levels may explain why women are more susceptible to migraines than males.

Some study indicates that when oestrogen levels rise and subsequently fall, blood vessel contractions may occur. This results in excruciating pain. According to other studies, oestrogen deficiency makes facial and scalp nerves more susceptible to pain.

What often causes migraine headaches?

Migraine sufferers may be able to pinpoint factors that appear to initiate the symptoms. Some examples of possible causes include:

• tension and other feelings

• biological and environmental factors, such as hormone fluctuations or exposure to light or odours

• fatigue and alterations in a person's sleep pattern

• glaring or flashing lights

• climate cjange

- specific foods and beverages

The American headache society advocates keeping a headache journal to record triggers. Bringing this information to your healthcare provider's attention enables him or her to find headache management solutions.

Chapter 6

Migraines diagnosis

Several people attempt to treat their migraines on their own, which can involve spending many hours in a dark, quiet room attempting to manage pain and other symptoms with otc drugs. The illness can go untreated for years, so depriving the individual of proper treatment.

Although some individuals use the terms "migraine" and "headache" interchangeably, a migraine is more than just a headache. Actually, it is a neurological disorder. A headache is typically one of the symptoms of a migraine episode, which also includes visual abnormalities, nausea, and vertigo.

If you experience frequent headaches and other migraine symptoms, it may be time to seek a diagnosis. In most cases, your primary care physician can evaluate your symptoms and determine the most effective treatment, but in some instances, you may be sent to a neurologist.

After receiving a migraine diagnosis, you can begin the necessary treatment.

Does it matter what type of headache or migraine i have?

Migraine sufferers may also experience various types of headache, which may require a different therapeutic strategy.

For instance, tension headaches may react to lifestyle modifications and alternative treatments. It is also possible to experience other types of headaches, such as tension headaches, concurrently with migraine.

A correct diagnosis will influence how it is treated. Menstrual or menstrually-related migraine, for instance, can be triggered by hormonal fluctuations during a woman's monthly cycle. On specific days of the month, preventive medication (a treatment meant to prevent or minimise the intensity of an attack) or a daily birth control tablet that may reduce hormonal swings may be used to treat this type of migraine.

How frequent or severe must my headaches be before I seek diagnosis?

Individuals who get migraines once or twice per month and are able to control them with over-the-counter medications such as ibuprofen have the option of seeking additional treatment.

If you experience headaches more than four times per month and they negatively influence your quality of life, you should consider obtaining a migraine diagnosis and treatment." Even those with less frequent migraine attacks, perhaps once or twice a month, who are incapacitating enough to need them to miss a whole day of work or be in bed all day should seek a diagnosis and medical therapy.

Chapter 7

Acute Migraine

Attacks of severe migraine are called acute.Acute migraines are commonly treated in hospital emergency rooms. About 3% of annual visits to the ED in the US are for headaches. There is evidence that treating this condition in the ED with opioids increases the likelihood of future visits, hospitalisation, and ED stays.

Acute migraines are often treated with opioids in the ER, despite the fact that published recommendations recommend nonopioid management.

Over the course of 14 months, there were 1,222 ED visits for acute migraines, and opioids were administered for 35.8% of those visits. Opioid prescriptions for acute migraine were written for a median of 7 days (interquartile range 4-20 days) at a median daily dosage of 22.5 mme, according to another study analysing medical claims data for privately insured persons in 2017.

frequency of prescriptions

In 36 percent of cases, emergency room patients under the age of 25 who presented with migraines were given an opioid prescription.

Substance abuse occurs too frequently and with too many drugs.

Dose of 22.5 mme over the course of 7 days

Opioids are often administered for 7 days at a median dosage of 22.5 mme for acute migraines.

For migraine sufferers, the best treatment options include the triptans (almotriptan, eletriptan, frovatriptan, naratriptan, rizatriptan, sumatriptan [oral, nasal spray, injectable, transcutaneous patch], zolmitriptan [oral and nasal spray], and dihydroergotamine (nasal spray, inhaler) (level a).

Nonspecific therapies such as acetaminophen, nonsteroidal anti-inflammatory drugs (NSAIDs; aspirin, diclofenac, ibuprofen, and naproxen), opioids (butorphanol nasal spray), sumatriptan/naproxen, and acetaminophen/aspirin/caffeine are useful (level a).

Several treatments for acute migraines have been shown to be effective. Clinicians need to consider pharmaceutical efficacy, potential side effects, and medication-related adverse events when prescribing acute medications for migraine. Opioids like butorphanol, codeine/acetaminophen, and tramadol/acetaminophen can be helpful, but they shouldn't be used on a regular basis.

A lack of evidence showing efficacy and concern over subacute or long-term side effects suggest that injectable morphine and hydromorphone should be avoided as first-line therapy.

The emergency room should administer intravenous metoclopramide, prochlorperazine, and subcutaneous sumatriptan to adults with acute migraine if they meet the criteria for these treatments.

Chapter 8

Migraine in children

If a kid under 12 years old presents with a headache and one or more "red flag" symptoms, they should be referred to a professional as soon as possible, as per guidelines from the National Institute for Health and Care Excellence (nice). Rapid diagnosis and treatment of intracranial pathology, such as a brain tumour, should be possible within a few hours at the latest.

Sometimes it's tough to tell if a kid has a migraine. In spite of the absence of external signs of trauma such blood, bruises, fever, or broken bones, the agony can be severe.

Sixty percent of young people get headaches at some point. Moreover, over 10% of young people endure the pain and disability of migraines. Migraine is a debilitating neurological disorder that can strike anyone at any time.

Children can experience migraines similarly to adults, although the symptoms may look different. When parents have a firm grasp on the condition, they are better prepared to aid their child in coping with triggers and exploring treatment options.

What signs and symptoms should parents look out for in a child with a migraine?

How can you know if your kid has a migraine or just a regular headache? Signs and symptoms vary from person to person. However, if you find yourself nodding in agreement with any of the following, it's possible that your child's headache is due to migraine and you should have them checked out.

Migraine headaches typically cause moderate to severe pain in the head. Unilateral, throbbing headaches are also possible. On the other hand, this is hardly ever the case with young people. In other cases, they may have a continuous, bilateral discomfort that is typically, but not always, situated in the temples or the area just above the eyes. Symptoms including nausea, vomiting, sensitivity to light, and sensitivity to sound are more common in youngsters after assaults but last much less time.

Some kids also complain of dizziness, blurred vision, and trouble focusing.

When an episode begins, some babies have severe stomach pain.

The headache is severe enough that the child will have to miss school and other commitments (or it keeps them from being at their best when they do those activities).

In exceedingly rare cases, a child's depression or irritability could be the result of migraine.

Some young people will see an aura before their migraines begin. Auras are a form of visual disturbance, though they can also impair speech or induce numbness in the face and arms.

The frequency of migraine attacks can be used to further classify the condition. Those who suffer from episodic migraine have a monthly headache frequency of less than 15 days on average. Chronic migraine sufferers get headaches on more than 15 days per month on average.

Why do kids have migraines?

There is a 50-75% chance that a child may develop migraines if one or both of the parents do. If younger generations know their family's medical history, especially if it involves migraine, they have a better chance of receiving an early and accurate diagnosis.

Most cases of migraine in children and adolescents occur without any warning. It was not their fault that they were attacked, either for doing or not doing anything. In most cases, this is how the condition manifests itself. There are clear triggers for some children's assaults. There are a few common factors that affect a large number of people, but each person has their own set of triggers. Common precipitating factors include weather, barometric pressure, hormonal shifts, concussions, traumatic brain traumas, and stress (both good and negative).

Women are more prone to suffer from migraines, and their first attack often coincides with menstruation. This disorder affects three times as many females as males. Despite their importance, the role of hormones in migraine is poorly understood.

When it comes to youngsters, how do we determine if they have a migraine?

Your child's head ache may be migraine, but a diagnosis cannot be made with a blood test or scan (ultrasound, ct scan, x-ray, or mri). The only method for your doctor to discover the reason of your child's head pain is to talk to your child about the specifics of their head pain, their response to current and prior treatments, their family history, and how their head pain affects their daily functioning and quality of life.

Most children and adolescents who suffer from migraines do not benefit from imaging. But there are times when it's best to get an MRI. When a child is under the age of three and experiencing headaches, imaging may be helpful if the child appears with a severe new headache type, shows headache-related symptoms including vision or swallowing issues, and demonstrates weakness or changes in gait. The results of a patient's physical examination can help a doctor decide if an MRI is necessary. Determine if and when a child with migraine needs imaging.

Children often develop concerns after learning they suffer migraines since the illness is unfamiliar. Prepare yourself for questions from your youngster regarding migraines.

What treatments are there for paediatric migraines?

Numerous approaches are typically used in the management of children's migraines. In general, raising healthy children is beneficial. Most doctors will start with informing patients' families about potentially helpful lifestyle changes for addressing headaches. Methods that contribute to this goal include maintaining a regular sleep schedule, preventing hunger between meals, increasing one's level of physical activity, drinking plenty of water, and controlling one's stress levels.

Another part of treating paediatric migraines is finding effective pain medications that may be given to children as soon as they experience the first symptoms. Acute medicine is what we call it. Achieving pain relief within an hour is a common goal, as is getting back to regular activities as soon as possible.

If a child has multiple attacks each week, the doctor may prescribe additional medicine to lessen the severity and frequency of the attacks. Drugs like amitriptyline and topiramate, as well as vitamins and minerals like magnesium and riboflavin, are sometimes given as prophylactic measures over the course of several months.

What can parents do to help their kid who keeps getting migraines?

Caring for a child who suffers from migraines requires constant and open communication to guarantee that everyone is on the same page and that the child is getting the right therapy.

Your child's migraines may be causing academic difficulties, as seen by frequent absences and low grades. The parental role is crucial. Keep an eye on your kid's grades and attendance and tell the school staff about his or her migraine. Your child's teachers and school nurses may learn more about migraines and how to accommodate students who suffer from them with your help.

If your child suffers from migraines, you should encourage him or her to be forthright about it with his or her friends. This may seem like a lot to ask, especially of older children, but it will be for the best in the long run. Find out how to help your child manage social situations, extracurricular activities, and daily routines when they suffer from migraines.

The American Migraine Foundation works to alleviate suffering for people who suffer from migraines. The most up-to-date information and news regarding paediatric migraine can be found at the AMF's centralised resource site. If you need help locating a doctor, use our find a doctor tool. As a group, we are as tenacious as a migraine.

Headaches in children are the same as in adults, albeit the specific symptoms may vary. The pain from a migraine in an adult often lasts at least four hours, but in a child it may subside sooner.

Especially in younger children who are unable to communicate their symptoms, it may be challenging to determine the type of headache in a child due to symptom distinctions. However, there does appear to be a correlation between the prevalence of specific symptoms and demographic factors.

Headaches brought on by migraines often result in

• Pain in the head that throbs or pulses

• Pain that worsens with motion

• Nausea

• Vomiting

• Pain in the belly

•Superior light and sound sensitivities

Even infants can get migraines. Small children who are unable to express their distress through words may cry or rock back and forth.

Migraine attacks triggered by tension

Tension headaches can result from a variety of factors.

Soreness that does not become worse with activity; mild to severe, asymmetrical stiffness in the head and neck muscles.

Nausea and vomiting are common side effects of migraine migraines.

Younger kids may pull back from regular play and want to nap more. Headaches caused by tension typically persist between 30 minutes and several days.

Headaches that come in clusters

Cluster headaches in kids under the age of 10 are quite unusual. On the whole, they: Usually happen in groups of five or more, with frequency ranging from once every other day to eight headaches a day.

Include sobbing, congestion, a runny nose, restlessness, or worry, and last fewer than three hours. The pain is intense and stabbing, and it's on one side of the head.

Professionals call migraines and tension headaches that occur more than 15 times per month "chronic daily headache" (cdh). Overuse of pain medications, especially over-the-counter ones, can lead to CdH. Infections and minor head injuries are also possible causes of this condition.

When should I see a doctor?

While most headaches are harmless, you should visit a doctor right away if your kid is experiencing any of the following symptoms:

Awaken your sleeping child

Decline or rise in occurrence

Sculpt your kid into a new person.

If someone is injured, especially if they take a blow to the head, it is important to provide first aid.

Changes in vision or persistent vomiting

Often accompanied by a high temperature, neck pain, or stiffness

If you are worried about your child's headaches or have any questions, it is best to talk to their doctor.

Infection and disease Common childhood headache triggers include colds, flu, ear infections, and sinus problems. Headaches are a rare symptom of meningitis or encephalitis.

Shock to the head

Getting a bump or bruise can result in a headache. If your child has fallen or been struck on the head forcefully, even though most head injuries are mild, you should take them to the hospital immediately. In addition, if your child's head pain persists after a head injury, it's important to see a doctor.

Effects on the Heart and Soul

Stress and anxiety, brought on by problems with friends, teachers, or parents, can lead to headaches in children. Depressed children may suffer from headaches, especially if they have trouble recognizing their own emotions of sadness and loneliness.

Behavioral traits that run in the family

Headaches and migraines tend to be hereditary. Nitrates, a food preservative found in bacon, bologna, and hot dogs, and the food additive msg have both been linked to an increase in headache complaints. Caffeine, which is found in beverages like soda, chocolate, and sports drinks, is another potential headache trigger.

Potential threats

In general, headaches can affect any kid, although they seem to occur more frequently in:

- Women when they hit menarche

- A higher risk exists for headaches and migraines in children who have a family history of these disorders.
- Teenagers in Their Late Teens

Prevention

The following may aid in preventing headaches or lessening their severity in children:

Adopt some healthy routines.

If your kid practices healthy habits, he or she may avoid future headaches. Get enough sleep, keep up your exercise routine, eat healthy meals and snacks, drink at least eight glasses of water every day, and cut back on your caffeine use are all examples of healthy lifestyle choices.

Decrease your worries

Stress and a busy schedule may raise the likelihood that you'll suffer from headaches. Watch out for signs that your kid might be experiencing stress, such slacking off at school or having problems making friends. Talking to a therapist could be helpful if you suspect that your child's headaches are the result of anxiety or depression.

Keep a record of your headaches.

Keeping a notebook can be helpful in identifying the source of your child's headaches. Track when the headache started, how long it lasted, and what helped.

Take note of how your kid responds to any painkillers you give him or her.

If you keep a headache diary for your child, you may get insight into his or her symptoms and be more equipped to take preventative measures.

Get rid of the things that are giving you headaches.

Do your best to stay away from any potential headache causes, such as caffeine. Keeping a headache diary for your child will help you figure out what triggers his or her migraines.

Do as your doctor tells you. If your child suffers from severe, daily headaches that cause significant impairment to daily life, his or her doctor may recommend prophylactic medicine. When taken at regular intervals, certain medications, such as antidepressants, anticonvulsants, and beta blockers, may lessen the frequency and severity of headaches. Headaches in children are the same as in adults, albeit the specific symptoms may vary. The pain from a migraine in an adult often lasts at least four hours, but in a child it may subside sooner.

Especially in younger children who are unable to communicate their symptoms, it may be challenging to determine the type of headache in a child due to symptom distinctions. However, there does appear to be a correlation between the prevalence of specific symptoms and demographic factors.

Even infants can get migraines. Small children who are unable to express their distress through words may cry or rock back and forth.

Younger children could become withdrawn from play and seek out more sleep. Headaches caused by tension typically persist between 30 minutes and several days.

Cluster headaches in kids under the age of 10 are quite unusual. On the whole, they: Usually happen in groups of five or more, with frequency ranging from once every other day to eight headaches a day. Be localized to one side of the head, last fewer than three hours, and feel like a combination of pins and needles and a severe headache.

If you are worried about your child's headaches or have any questions, it is best to talk to their doctor.

Your child's headaches could be caused by a number of factors. Examples of this are:

Infection and disease Common childhood headache triggers include colds, flu, ear infections, and sinus problems. Headaches are a rare symptom of meningitis or encephalitis.

Chapter 9

MIGRAINE AND STRESS

Different from headaches, migraines are not widely understood to have a cause. However, there are recognized triggers, such as stress.

The American headache society reports that stress is a migraine trigger in roughly 4 out of 5 cases. Another potential migraine trigger has been discovered as relaxation after a time of severe stress.

What do the studies reveal?

Scientist speculate that serotonin levels in the brain may fluctuate as a result of migraines. Serotonin aids in controlling pain.

Researchers think that even more than stress itself, relaxing following periods of intense stress can cause migraines. The "let-down" effect is the name given to this.

Some claim that this effect is related to other illnesses, including the flu or a cold.

Migraine signs and symptoms

It's likely that you'll have stress symptoms before migraine symptoms at first. Typical signs of stress include:

- Uneasy stomach
- Skeletal tension
- Irritability
- Fatigue
- A chest ache
- Quick heartbeat
- Depression and sadness
- Absence of sex desire

A day or two before the migraine itself, symptoms may start to appear. The prodrome stage is what it is termed. These could be signs of this stage:

- Fatigue
- Cravings for food
- Mood shifts
- Neck rigidity
- Constipation

❖ Often yawning

A migraine with aura is a condition that some people suffer following the prodrome stage. Auras can interfere with vision. It can also result in issues with movement, speech, and sensation in some persons, such as:

Observing bright dots, forms, or flashing lights

The face, arms, or legs tingling

Having trouble speaking

Transient eyesight loss

The attack phase of a headache is when the pain first manifests. If untreated, the attack hase symptoms can extend for a few hours to a few days. Each person's symptoms are different in intensity.

Some signs could be:

A sensitivity to light and sound

Heightened sensitivity to touch and scent

Throbbing head ache in the front, back, temples, or on one or both sides of your head

Nausea

Vomiting

Dizziness

Feeling dizzy or ill at ease

The postdrome phase is the last stage. It might lead to mood swings ranging from exhilaration and a very cheerful feeling to fatigue and feeling worn out. Also possible is a dull headache. Typically, these symptoms last for 24 hours.

How to stop migraines brought on by stress

Medication is used in the treatment of migraines to alleviate symptoms and stop further attacks. Finding measures to lessen your stress will help you avoid additional attacks if stress is what's triggering your migraines.

Medications

Among the medications used to treat migraine pain are:

Otc painkillers, such as acetaminophen (aleve, motrin) or ibuprofen (advil, motrin) (tylenol)

Acetaminophen, aspirin, and caffeine-containing over-the-counter migraine drugs like excedrin migraine triptans like rizatriptan, almotriptan, and sumatriptan (imitrex) (maxalt) ergots, such as cafergot and migergot, which mix ergotaminc and caffeine.

If you experience nausea and vomiting along with a migraine, you might also be prescribed anti-nausea medicine.

In the treatment of severe migraines, corticosteroids are occasionally used with other drugs. Due to the negative side effects, frequent use is not advised.

Preventive medicine may be right for you if:

At least four of your severe bouts occur each month, attacks that last longer than 12 hours happen to you.

Medication for pain relief doesn't help you.

You go through extended episodes of numbness or aura.

To lessen the frequency, duration, and intensity of your migraines, preventive drugs are used daily or once a month.

If stress is a recognized migraine trigger, your doctor may advise taking the medicine only during periods of extreme stress, such as the days before a demanding work week or important event.

Preventive drugs consist of:

Propranolol is one example of a beta-blocker. Drugs that inhibit calcium channels, like verapamil (calan, verelan)

Antidepressants like venlafaxine and amitriptyline (effexor xr)

Antagonists of the cgrp receptor, such as erenumab-aooe (aimovig)

Naproxen (naprosyn), a prescription anti-inflammatory drug, can help prevent migraines and lessen their effects.

However, it has been discovered that anti-inflammatories raise the risk of heart attacks, stomach ulcers, and bleeding. It's not advised to use it frequently.

Alternative therapies

You can take a few steps to reduce your risk of developing a migraine due to stress. These things might also aid in reducing migraine and stress-related symptoms. Think about the following:

Include relaxation techniques like yoga and meditation in your everyday practice.

Get enough sleep, which you can do by maintaining a regular bedtime each night.

Try getting a massage. According to a 2006 study, it can help prevent migraines, lower cortisol levels, and lower anxiety.

Workout more often lessen stress and possibly aid in preventing let-down migraines following a stressful time.

Consult your doctor if you're having problems managing your stress or if you discover that stress is a migraine trigger. They may offer suggestions for reducing stress.

How to deal with stress as a migraine trigger

It would be an understatement to say that managing migraine's persistent discomfort is difficult. When stress is one of your migraine triggers, those difficulties are amplified. Chronic pain increases stress, which in turn increases the risk of migraines. And to top it all off, if your body is used to constant stress, taking the weekend off can cause a "let down" migraine when your stress levels suddenly drop. Not exactly a win-win situation for migraine sufferers.

Establish your priorities

Consider your priorities and make two lists with the headings "life" and "now." what items on your list are the most crucial? What can you take away? When planning your time and assigning priorities to your tasks, keep the vital things in mind. Being constantly on the run and concentrating on things that make you unhappy is not the ideal strategy for living a low-stress lifestyle.

Save your time

Recognize when you need to make time for yourself. Remember that your needs matter and use your schedule defensively. Schedule a half-hour during the day for yourself, and utilize it to get up and move around. If you're a stay-at-home parent, think about hiring a cheap mother's helper or sitter to play with your kids at your house during the day so you can relax.

Schedule relationships and personal development time

According to studies, conversing with others reduces stress. Plan "together time" with your partner, and make a conscious effort to get up from the couch and do something enjoyable. Engage your network of supporters and extend your support to others. Stress can be immediately reduced by boosting interpersonal interaction and giving priority to the things that make you joyful.

Develop your communication and assertiveness

It's likely that you aren't letting people know what you want from life if you communicate passively. You may lessen your stress level, express yourself clearly, speak without becoming angry, and acquire more self-confidence by having effective communication skills. A free assertiveness training course can teach you how to express your needs and wants.

Obtained enough sleep

Over 85% of the participants in a recent study of over 200 migraine sufferers showed clinically significant poor sleep quality, which is linked to headache frequency, sadness, and anxiety.

Sleep improvement strategy

Exercise on a daily basis, abstaining from food and caffeine before bed, going to bed at the same time every night, and avoiding devices for 30 minutes to an hour before bedtime are all examples of good sleep hygiene.

It's stressful enough to manage migraine symptoms; there's no need to deal with additional outside variables. By making the necessary changes in your life, you might potentially lessen additional migraine symptoms. Start moving in the correct way right now.

Control your migraines and their causes.

For many people, stress is a frequent migraine cause. Consider strategies to maintain your workplace as stress-free as you can if this is the case for you. Project and time management strategies that space out deadlines and reduce the constant stream of updates from your inbox and other programmes are one method to do this. Other strategies include keeping your workstation comfortable, installing an anti-glare screen on your computer, purchasing an ergonomic chair, and taking periodic breaks outside. The most important thing is to keep a migraine first aid kit at your workplace. Pack a bottle of water, some snacks, your migraine medication, and a cold forehead pack.

Do something

Tell your designated advocate as soon as you start to sense an attack coming on so you can collaborate to carry out the pre-determined plan for returning home safely. Whatever your coping tactics, it is advised to take your medication as soon as possible before switching to other tested methods that can be particular to your symptoms. Take a taxi, get a lift from a friend, or your workplace advocate to get home. Avoid using public transit and don't drive. Driving while suffering from a migraine attack can be quite dangerous.

Being depressed, unhappy, or blue may not always occur at the same time as a migraine for some people. Actually, three to four of every ten migraine sufferers will also be sad. Therefore, depression is rather typical among migraine sufferers. Unfortunately, this can make managing migraines more difficult.

But why are migraine sufferers more likely to experience depression? Here are a few options:

Your ancestry

Since migraines and depression frequently run in families, this may be a contributing factor. However, it doesn't provide the complete story because not every member of a family may experience migraines or depression.

Being in pain increases your risk of depression. This seems logical given that it is easy to feel as though things aren't going to get any better the longer and more frequently you experience migraines. However, there are some people who were depressed before they developed headaches, and there are others who have long experienced migraines but are not depressed.

How your brain interprets data. Your brain does not process information precisely the same as other people's brains if you suffer from migraines, depression, or both. Because of this, your doctor may recommend medicine to assist restore mental equilibrium.

Additionally, your doctor may discuss with you daily activities and lifestyle modifications that can help reduce your risk of developing migraines and improve your mood.

Ask your doctor whether they might be able to help you with your mood and your migraines if you are generally down or don't enjoy things as much as you once did.

Do you ever experience a pounding headache and achy jaw in the morning?

Your temporomandibular joint (TMJ) and the muscles around the joint that are linked to clenching and grinding may be to blame for this migraine. The lower jaw's (mandible) joint with the temporal bone is where the TMJ is situated.

Clenching, grinding, and the onset or triggering of headaches are strongly correlated. The clicking of the joint, discomfort, swelling, locking, and trouble chewing can all be symptoms of joint pain. Additionally, the back, neck, head, and ears may experience pain.

Stress is probably a factor that causes people to clench their teeth while they are awake. This frequently occurs when people are tense, annoyed, or trying to concentrate. Trauma can occasionally cause jaw pain.

Chewing gum contributes significantly to TMJ pain. Most individuals are unaware of the harm that constant gum chewing causes. The equivalent of chewing gum all day would be performing bicep curls. You would get bicep pain. Your jaw would also feel the wear and tear of this unending activity.

Migraines and TMJ symptoms frequently coexist, making it challenging to tell the difference between the two. Each one can be making the other painful condition worse. Due to heredity and hormones, women are more likely than males to experience headaches and tmj pain.

The discomfort can be reduced with the help of a number of treatments. The easiest fixes involve changing one's way of life. Avoid chewing on your lips, cheeks, pencils, or fingernails. The jaw can get more stressed even if you just hold the phone up to your head. Avoid eating sticky, crunchy foods and chewing gum. Don't consume an entire apple in one mouthful. Sandwiches and hamburgers in pieces. Try not to open your mouth too wide. While yawning, narrow the diameter of your mouth opening. Holding your face neutrally while relaxing your teeth and keeping them apart might also be beneficial. Exercises that gently extend your jaw can greatly improve your mood.

You have no control over clenching while you sleep. You will clench as you sleep if you have a clenching tendency. In order to prevent you from clenching or grinding your teeth while you sleep, dentists can create stabilising equipment (splints and nightguards) just for you. The use of over-the-counter appliances is not advised. These "do-it-yourself" solutions frequently don't produce a suitable fit and frequently make you clench more. They may also be extremely painful.

In addition to stress, other more severe problems including joint degeneration, arthritis, or inflammation might also be present. Preventing the TMJ disease from getting worse is crucial.

TMJ has to be examined if you have severe jaw pain in the morning. One possible cause of your morning headache is TMJ. Between 4 and 9 a.m., almost half of all migraines are recorded. A regular morning migraine is unusual. Recurrent morning headaches of the migraine variety are frequently brought on by overnight withdrawal from an abused medicine. OSA, which is underdiagnosed, is another contributing factor.

Obstructive snoring (OSA)

One of the telltale indicators of OSA is waking up frequently with headaches and feeling unrefreshed. People who with sleep apnea experience severe daytime weariness. Snoring, headaches in the morning, difficulty concentrating, anxiety, depression, elevated blood pressure, and gastric reflux are some typical OSA symptoms. OSA can affect people of any size, despite the typical OSA sufferer being overweight. A polysomnogram, a sleep study that is performed at a sleep centre, is used to formally diagnose sleep apnea. Since they are becoming more and more accessible, you might request a sleep study at home.

In OSA, the upper airway is either completely or partially closed while you sleep. Breathing pauses are caused by a restricted, occluded, or floppy airway. Snoring may stop by sleeping on one's side. This most frequently occurs while doing so while lying on one's back. Sleeping on one's back may be avoided by using several kinds of "sleep blocks". Even while the majority of us occasionally snore, it is neither normal or healthy to do so frequently.

The most typical therapy for severe OSA is a face mask that is given by a doctor. Applying continuous positive airway pressure is this device (cpap). With the large gadget and its impact on breathing, many people have problems falling asleep. Compared to either the large mask or cpap, dental mandibular advancement appliances are often easier to endure. Dental appliances can be equally as beneficial for mild to moderate OSA.

Major and severe health implications can result from untreated sleep apnea. A lack of oxygen to the brain is repeatedly experienced by the patient, increasing their chance of developing conditions like cardiovascular disease, congestive heart failure, high blood pressure, stroke, diabetes, depression, weight gain, and obesity. According to "science daily," those with untreated OSA have a 30% higher probability of dying from a heart attack or another type of cardiovascular disease. Due to the morphology of their noses, mouths, and necks as well as their stature, more men than women are likely to have OSA.

Those who live in areas with harsh winters and a lot of snow appreciate the transformation from winter to spring. However, for the proportion of migraineurs who also have asthma, hay fever, or allergies, this is the time of year when headaches tend to worsen and are accompanied by the signs of seasonal allergens.

Chapter 10

Non-pharmacological approaches to the treatment of headaches in children and adolescents

Headache disorders are prevalent in children and adolescents, affecting up to 88% of the pediatric and teenage population, with 6% experiencing persistent headaches. Headache can cause severe handicap, including lost school days and restrictions on extracurricular activities such as social gatherings with peers, family gatherings, and sports. In general, non steroidal anti-inflammatory medications (nsaids), analgesics, and triptans constitute the pharmacological treatment for acute bouts. As with adults, proper administration is required for efficacy, with a particular focus on providing information about the danger of medication overuse headache.

Antiepileptics, such as topiramate, are regarded as first-line treatment for migraine prevention, and some medicines used to prevent migraines in adults are frequently prescribed for children. Particularly relevant side effects for children and adolescents include weight loss or increase, paresthesias, cognitive slowdown, and tiredness. Due to the increased risk of developing polycystic ovarian syndrome as well as the potential teratogenic consequences of several of these substances, adolescents must exercise caution. However, drug treatment is not always necessary, and preventive medication is not the first line of defence in the great majority of instances. In recent years, non-pharmacological treatments for headache disorders, primarily those that are cognitive, behavioural, or psychophysiological in character, as well as non-invasive neurostimulation, have received growing attention. In terms of reductions in the frequency of headaches, the aforementioned treatments have been shown to have substantial improvements, often ranging from 35 to 50%. However, the majority of published studies on non-pharmacological treatments have been conducted on adults, and current literature reviews have not focused significantly on young patients with headaches. The purpose of this review is to assist address this deficiency by giving current information on more recent investigations of non-pharmacological approaches to the treatment of headaches in children and adolescents.

Relaxation techniques

The aforementioned methods can prevent migraine, but cannot treat them. There are fortunately various non pharmaceutical therapy choices.

First, there are relaxing techniques. Since stress is a typical migraine trigger, relaxation training can be an effective treatment.

In relaxation techniques, deep breathing and progressive muscular relaxation are employed. To execute deep breathing exercises, one must visualize a place right below the navel and breathe into it, filling the stomach with air. Once the abdomen is full, slowly exhale all the air, and you should begin to feel more relaxed with each exhalation.

Progressive muscular relaxation is quite unique. At this point, you must shift your focus to your breathing. You still need to take a few deep breaths and exhale slowly, but this time you're conducting a mental scan of your body.

By rotating the head twice in a smooth, circular motion, patients suffering from a migraine can instantly relax the tight areas. Then, roll the shoulders forth and backward numerous times, allowing the muscles to rest for several minutes while recalling a nice idea.

This technique may, with practice, not only lessen the frequency of migraines but also enhance stress management.

Exercise

Exercise is another option, though it can be both a migraine trigger and a therapy, so it must be performed appropriately.

Patients who suffer from migraines should not begin an exercise routine without warming up for five to ten minutes first. Those who are new to physical activity should begin with easy exercises such as yoga, strolling, and swimming until they become adapted.

By lowering tension, regular exercise can reduce the frequency or intensity of headaches.

Acupuncture

Acupuncture involves the insertion of five to twenty extremely thin needles at various locations on the skin, which is believed to restore the flow of qi. While the needles are in the body, the practitioner may apply heat and gently rotate them. In the majority of instances, the needles are left in place for 10 to 20 minutes while the patient relaxes.

Pain is the most prevalent indication for acupuncture, as it enhances the body's natural painkillers and promotes blood flow. The American headache society recently endorsed acupuncture for migraines, and research indicate that acupuncture helps reduce migraine pain and frequency.

Sleep

Last but not least, it is essential to get sufficient sleep. Migraine sufferers typically awaken fatigued and have difficulty falling asleep.

The national sleep foundation suggests that the average adult sleep between 7 and 9 hours per night. Studies have demonstrated a correlation between sleep deprivation and both the frequency and severity of migraines.

As a result, many people with migraines suffer from sleeplessness, which can lead to a vicious cycle that contributes to recurrent migraine headaches. Good sleep hygiene, such as avoiding daytime naps, not eating before night, and maintaining a regular bedtime, can solve this issue.

Migraines are a persistent annoyance, but adopting the appropriate precautions can reduce their frequency and severity. It is essential for patients to take care of themselves and ensure that they are getting enough sleep and exercise.

If migraines are persistent and recurrent, patients should speak with their physician about combining pharmaceutical and non pharmacological therapy. These tips should help not only migraines, but overall health as well.

Headache treatments

Several methods, including lower cervical intramuscular injections, nerve blocks, pericranial injections, and onabotulinumtoxina (botox) injections, have showed efficacy in migraine management. Although the mechanism of action for headache treatments is unknown, it has been demonstrated that these treatments lessen migraine frequency and intensity. All of these operations can be performed in the clinic, and the sphenopalatine ganglion block can be administered at home as needed.

If migraines are not improving, it may be necessary to seek less common drugs. Inhibitors of monoamine oxidase, stimulants, steroids, and atypical analgesics are examples (eg, ketamine). Despite the risks and difficulties associated with these drugs, they can be used as part of a strategy to transform failure into success.

Chapter 11

Monitor Migraine

Migraine apps are a fantastic method to monitor migraine triggers, communicate data with your physician, and keep extensive records of headache episodes, all of which can provide extra insight into triggers and how to avoid them. These migraine apps may help your doctor assess the sort of headache you experience and the best effective medication by identifying patterns.

Migraine monitor app is more than just an intuitive tool for tracking your headaches, their severity, duration, and triggers; it also gives you access to the support of your doctor (or our headache navigator) and a community of anonymous headache sufferers with whom you can interact, if you so choose. Reports that are simple to read can be shared with family, friends, and your doctor.

Receive daily information, such as news, suggestions, and inspirations, that will help you control your headaches.